I0700849

COUPLES MASSAGE

The Complete Guide To Couples Massage Guide: Understanding The Tradition, Technique, And Transformative Healing

BANABAS WISDOM

Copyright © 2023 By Banabas Wisdom

All Rights Reserved

Contents

Introductory 5

CHAPTER ONE 8

A Variety Of Couples Massage
Techniques....................................8

Distinction From Individual Massage ...13

CHAPTER TWO 19

The Critical Value Of Communication ..19

Setting Up For The Massage 26

CHAPTER THREE 34

Fundamental Massage Techniques 34

Methods Of Acquiring Connection.......41

CHAPTER FOUR 49

Individualizing Massages For One
Another..49

The Utilization Of Aromatherapy........56

CHAPTER FIVE 63

Management Of Frequent Obstacles ...63

Suggestions For An Effective Couples
Massage 70

CHAPTER SIX **78**

  **Expert Assistance And Continuing
Education** **78**

  Summary...**86**

THE END **90**

Introductory

A Couples Massage is a form of massage therapy in which two individuals receive massages from their respective massage therapists simultaneously while in the same room. A couples massage aims to provide an opportunity for family members, acquaintances, or partners to partake in the therapeutic experience in a communal area.

Spas and massage therapy centers frequently provide couples massages, which can serve as a therapeutic and unifying experience for the two people participating. By harmonizing their techniques and movements, the massage therapists can guarantee that both clients enjoy a synchronized and harmonious experience.

In addition to stress relief and relaxation, couples massage provides an opportunity to spend precious time together in a tranquil and calming setting. It can serve as a means for family members to share a spa day, a romantic outing for couples, or a way for peers to strengthen their bonds.

Couples massages may be tailored to the specific requirements and preferences of each participant, whether they favor a soothing, relaxing touch or a stimulating, therapeutic approach.

CHAPTER ONE
A Variety Of Couples Massage Techniques

Couples massages are customizable to accommodate the inclinations and requirements of the participants. A couples massage session may encompass the integration of a multitude of massage styles and techniques. The following are prevalent types of couples massage:

• Swedish massage consists of lengthy, flowing strokes, circular movements, and kneading; it is a soothing and tranquil technique. Its dual purpose is to enhance circulation and induce relaxation.

• Deep Tissue Massage: This technique targets connective tissue and deeper muscle layers. Consistently employed to treat chronic pain and specific muscle tension, it may be more intense than Swedish massage.

• Hot Stone Massage: To soothe and relax muscles, hot stones are applied to specific points on the body. In addition to massaging the body with the stones, the massage therapist may do so in order to provide a therapeutic and relaxing experience.

• Aromatherapy Massage: To enhance the massage experience, aromatherapy utilizes essential oils. An assortment of oils possess distinct properties that can induce relaxation, elevate the mood, or alleviate muscular tension.

• Thai massage consists of rhythmic movements, compression, and assisted flexibility. On a mat on the floor, it is typically performed with participants attired in comfortable apparel.

• Sports massage focuses primarily on the treatment of muscle strains and injuries. In addition to deep tissue techniques and stretching, additional therapeutic methods may be utilized.

• Shiatsu massage, which has its roots in Japan, utilizes targeted pressure on particular anatomical locations to facilitate the circulation of energy. The recipient is not required to be completely clothed during the procedure, and it frequently consists of joint mobilization and stretching.

• An Ayurvedic Couples Massage: An ancient Indian medical system, Ayurveda. Ayurvedic massage may incorporate the application of heating oils and distinct techniques that are customized to the dosha (constitution) of the individual.

It is crucial to inform the massage therapists of your preferences, any particular areas of concern, and the desired level of pressure when reserving a couples massage. This practice guarantees that the massage is tailored to accommodate the unique requirements of each recipient and elevates the overall ambiance.

Distinction From Individual Massage

The fundamental distinction between an individual massage and a couples massage is the environment and the quantity of participants during the treatment. The following are several fundamental differentiations:

• A couples massage entails the simultaneous provision of massages to two individuals within the confines of the same chamber.

It is a communal experience in which family, colleagues, or partners can all benefit from massage.

An solitary massage, on the other hand, is performed on a single recipient.

• Couples massage participants have the option of being situated in the same room or distinct rooms, contingent upon their personal preferences and level of comfort. During individual massages, the recipient generally occupies a private chamber.

• Synchronized Massage: The practitioners of couples massage may harmonize their strokes in order to provide both clients with a harmonious and synchronized experience. This coordination enhances the shared experience and imparts a unique quality to the session.

•   Shared   Relaxation   and camaraderie: Couples massages are frequently regarded as a form of camaraderie. It affords couples, acquaintances, and family members the chance to unwind and partake in a serene experience collectively. In contrast, individual massages are more tailored to the therapeutic and relaxation requirements of the recipient.

• Individual and couples massages are capable of being tailored to the particular   inclinations   and requirements of the recipients. However, therapists may need to consider the preferences of two individuals and modify the session accordingly during a couples massage.

• Communication is an essential aspect of both types of massages; however, in the context of a couples massage, there may be an additional dimension of communication between the participants. Individuals may opt to participate in a conversation, appreciate the massage in private company, or express their preferences to the therapists.

- Couples massages are frequently associated with an intimate or amorous environment, which contributes to their widespread appeal among couples seeking to share meaningful moments together.

The romantic aspect may encompass unique environmental elements, such as calming music or candlelight, which serve to augment the overall ambiance.

Although the fundamental tenets of massage therapy remain consistent, a couples massage is distinguished from individual massages by virtue of its context and the inherent enjoyment that couples derive from the session. Therapeutic benefits, stress relief, and relaxation are all potential benefits of both varieties of massage, which are customized to the individual preferences of each recipient.

CHAPTER TWO
The Critical Value Of Communication

Communication is essential in the context of massage therapy, regardless of whether a couple or an individual is receiving the treatment. Several factors underscore the significance of effective communication throughout a massage session:

1. Adaptation to the Individual Massage:

• By expressing your preferences, including desired pressure level, specific areas of concentration, and any distress or pain you may be experiencing, you enable the massage therapist to customize the session according to your unique requirements.

• Both partners should express their preferences during a couples massage in order to guarantee that the experience is pleasurable and fulfills the expectations of all parties involved.

2. Comfort and Security:

• It is imperative that you apprise the massage therapist of any pre-existing health conditions, injuries, or concerns that may affect your safety and overall well-being throughout the session.

• Should you experience any discomfort during the massage, including but not limited to the illumination, room temperature, or pressure level, please inform the therapist so that appropriate modifications can be implemented to guarantee your comfort.

3. Observations Made Throughout the Massage:

• Issuance of feedback throughout the massage is beneficial. In the event that the pressure is excessively intense or insufficiently profound, the therapist is able to make adjustments in real time to optimize your experience.

• Partners can engage in communication with one another and the clinicians during a couples massage to ensure mutual comfort and satisfaction throughout the session.

4. Psychological and Emotional Comfort:

• There are emotional and psychological benefits to massage therapy. The act of expressing any concerns or emotional reactions enables the therapist to establish an atmosphere that is both encouraging and soothing.

• During a couples massage, participants may opt to engage in conversation regarding their massage experience, thereby cultivating a feeling of camaraderie and mutual relaxation.

5. Consent by Informed Parties:

• Frequently, prior to the commencement of the massage, the therapist will discuss the massage plan and any particular techniques that will be employed. Consensus can be obtained and information conveyed through transparent communication regarding the proposed approach.

6. The adaptation of methodologies:

- Massage therapists possess a diverse range of techniques in their training. By expressing your inclinations towards a specific style or technique, the therapist is able to tailor the session in a way that aligns with your objectives and anticipations.

7. Pragmatic and Relaxation-Improving Factors:

- Efficient communication has the potential to foster a state of mental relaxation throughout the massage. Acquiring bodily awareness and communicating one's requirements promotes a mindful encounter, thereby augmenting the holistic advantages of the massage.

Bear in mind that communication that is candid and open is a reciprocal process. Active participation is required from both the massage therapist and the recipient to guarantee a positive and beneficial experience.

Effective communication among the partners and the therapists is a significant factor in creating a mutually pleasurable and shared experience during a couples massage.

Setting Up For The Massage

Preparing for a massage contributes to your comfort and satisfaction during the session. The following suggestions will assist you in preparing for your massage, be it a couple's or individual session:

1. Interactions with the Massage Practitioner:

• It is advisable to inform the massage therapist of any health concerns, injuries, or specific bodily areas that necessitate attention either during the initial consultation or prior to the commencement of the session.

• Please articulate your inclinations with respect to the pressure level, oil or lotion usage, and specific massage techniques that you find most favorable.

2. Regarding hygiene:

• Prior to the massage, ensure that you are spotless and refreshed by taking a shower or bath.

• Strong fragrances and colognes should be avoided, as they may disrupt the massage experience.

3. Clothing:

• I recommend visiting the retreat or massage therapy center while dressed comfortably. If necessary, a robe or disposable undergarments may be made available to you.

• Some massage styles, such as Thai massage, may require the practitioner to remain completely clothed; therefore, loose, comfortable clothing is recommended.

4. Regarding timing:

• It is advisable to be punctual for your appointment in order to foster an atmosphere of leisure and deceleration.

o If it is a couples massage, arrange to appear at the same time as your partner.

5.Sufficient hydration:

To remain hydrated, consume water before and after your massage. Toxins can be eliminated from the muscles through massage, and sufficient hydration can aid in their elimination.

6.Meditation and relaxation:

Prior to the massage, take a few moments to unwind and clear your mind. Meditation or deep breathing can assist in calming the nervous system and enhancing the experience as a whole.

To reduce distractions, power down your phone or place it in silent mode.

7.Accessory and Jewelry:

Inocrust the therapist's work by removing jewelry and accessories prior to the massage to prevent any potential interference.

Please store any valuable items in a locker or another designated area that the facility will provide.

8.Expectations Regarding Couples Massage:

Before undergoing a couples massage, you and your companion should discuss your expectations and preferences. This includes specific preferences regarding shared or private accommodations, as well as any desired amenities or features, such as aromatherapy or music.

9.Pre-Massage Strategies:

Proceed with planning your timetable subsequent to the massage. Afterward, it is frequently advantageous to arrange a period of relaxation as opposed to returning to a hectic schedule immediately.

10. As a gratuity:

• Please ensure to bring cash or a credit card to cover gratuity, unless the spa's policies specify otherwise.

It is imperative to emphasize the significance of communication, both with the massage therapist and your companion during a couples massage.

The greater the therapist's awareness of your preferences and particular concerns, the more effectively they can customize the massage to suit your requirements.

By following these methods, you can maximize the benefits of your massage and achieve optimal results.

CHAPTER THREE
Fundamental Massage Techniques

Various techniques of massage may be utilized on various areas of the body, contingent upon the objectives of the massage and the personal inclinations of the recipient. The following are fundamental massage techniques that massage therapists frequently employ:

1. Effleurage mechanisms:

• Long, expansive strokes are employed to prepare the muscles for a more intense massage by warming them up.

This methodology entails applying light to moderate pressure while gliding the hands across the epidermis.

2. Petrissage entails:

• Kneading and compression exercises encompass actions such as rolling, compressing, or pressing the muscles. Petrissage is frequently employed for circulation enhancement and tension release.

3. The frictional force:

• Utilize circular or transverse motions utilizing the palms, fingertips, or thumbs to generate thermal energy and disrupt muscle adhesions. Friction serves as a practical means of mitigating localized tension.

4. Tapotement is defined as:

• The utilization of rhythmic striking or percussive movements, such as hacking, pounding, and cupping. Tapotement is a revitalizing technique that aids in the release of tension and improvement of blood flow.

5. Regarding vibration:

• The user executes precise, swift trembling or swaying motions utilizing their fingertips or palms.

Vibration is frequently employed to promote relaxation and muscle soreness.

6. The compression process:

• Consistent application of pressure with the hands, palms, or fingers on a designated area. Trigger points can be released and muscle tension reduced through compression.

7. The stretch:

• Stretching muscles and joints gently can enhance range of motion and flexibility. Stretching is a frequently integrated component of massage, specifically in techniques such as Thai massage.

8. Joint Activation:

• The massage therapist executes passive joint movements with the intention of enhancing joint flexibility and diminishing rigidity. This is frequently employed alongside additional massage modalities.

9. Release of the Myofascial Tissue:

• By applying slow, sustained pressure to the fascia, which is a type of connective tissue, restrictions can be released and energy flow can be improved. A common application of myofascial release is to treat chronic tension and discomfort.

10. Point-of-trigger therapy:

• Through the application of sustained pressure to particular trigger points in the muscles, pain and tension can be alleviated. Frequently, this method is applied to specific regions of distress.

11. Fiber-to-Fiber Friction:

• By utilizing specific pressure along the muscle fibers, scar tissue and adhesions can be eliminated. Cross-fiber friction has the potential to facilitate tissue regeneration and aid in the treatment of injuries.

It is crucial to acknowledge that the selection of massage techniques is contingent upon a multitude of factors, encompassing the client's inclinations, the objectives of the massage, and any particular ailments or concerns that require attention.

Furthermore, proficient massage therapists frequently employ a blend of these methodologies in order to design an individualized massage regimen that is both efficacious and personalized.

Please do not hesitate to communicate with your therapist regarding your preferences, areas of concern, or distress while receiving a massage.

Methods Of Acquiring Connection

In the context of fostering a sense of connection during communal experiences such as couples massages, the integration of particular techniques has the potential to augment the overall rapport between participants. Listed below are some methods for fostering connection:

1. Intentional Breathing:

• Commence the exercise by engaging in a brief period of deliberate respiration collectively.

Slowly exhale and inhale while timing your breath with that of your companion. This not only facilitates relaxation but also creates a synchronized cadence.

2. Conscious Presence:

• Motivate both parties to experience complete presence in the present moment. Concentrate on the emotions, sounds, and sensations encountered throughout the massage. The connection is strengthened through the focus of mindful presence on the shared experience.

3. Synchronization of Physical Motions:

• A couple's massage should incorporate synchronized movements. Promote a harmonious and interconnected flow by encouraging both individuals to move or switch positions concurrently, provided that they are both at ease.

4. Nonverbal Modes of Communication:

• Employ non-verbal signals or gentle touches as means of conveying comfort or pleasure. This may be accomplished with a gentle squeeze of the hand or a reassuring palm placed on the shoulder. A sense of connection is strengthened through nonverbal communication.

5. Setting of Shared Intentions:

• Prior to the massage, engage in a conversation and establish mutual intentions. This may encompass objectives related to tension relief, relaxation, or simply devoting quality time together. By aligning intentions, a unified focus can be established.

6. Express Appreciation:

• One should pause either prior to or following the massage to convey appreciation to one another. Exhibit your gratitude regarding the experience and one another. Gratitude serves to amplify positive emotions and fortify the emotional bond.

7. Dialogue Encountered During the Massage:

• During the session, if you feel at ease, share your experience with one another and the massage therapists. Real-time discussion of the sensations or preferences serves to augment the communal aspect of the experience.

8. Muscular Relaxation Methods:

• Incorporate joint relaxation techniques that involve the active participation of both individuals. This may encompass companion stretches, synchronized breathing exercises, or gentle joint movements.

9. Committed Rituals:

• Incorporate communal rituals or procedures into the experience. This could involve a particular sequence of events preceding or following the massage, such as an intimate exchange of silence or a straightforward hand gesture.

10. After-Massage Contemplation:

• Following the massage, pause for a brief period of collective reflection. Elucidate on the emotions evoked by the experience and the aspect that brought you the most pleasure. Exchange of reflections fosters a stronger bond and generates a favorable recollection.

11. Develop a Congenial Ambiance:

• It is imperative to establish a massage environment that fosters connection. This could be accomplished through the use of aromatherapy, calming music, or illumination adjustments. An inviting and comfortable environment enriches the overall experience.Bear in mind that being attuned to one another's comfort levels and preferences is crucial.

By accommodating the particular dynamics of the participants, these methods can be modified to foster a stronger sense of connection throughout the experience.

CHAPTER FOUR
Individualizing Massages For One Another

In the context of a romantic setting, individualizing massages for one another can be an enjoyable and private experience. The subsequent advice will assist you in personalizing massages for your partner:

1. The Art of Communication:

- Commence the dialogue by considering one another's inclinations, any points of contention, and the ideal degree of intensity. Effective communication is crucial for ensuring that the massage is both pleasurable and customized to meet the specific requirements of each individual.

2. Selection of Methodologies:

• I would suggest integrating a variety of massage techniques in accordance with the preferences of your companion. While certain people may find solace in relaxed techniques and delicate strokes, others may have a preference for more intense and therapeutic pressure.

3. Concentrate on issue areas:

• Inquire with your companion regarding any particular areas of their body that may require additional attention. This may pertain to a specific muscle group characterized by persistent tension or an area afflicted with chronic pain.

4. Employing Lotions or Oils:

• Do not hesitate to inquire about your partner's oil or lotion preferences. As an aromatherapy option, perfumed oils may appeal to some individuals more than unscented alternatives. Ascertain that the selected product is appropriate for the skin type of your partner.

5. Thermostat and surroundings:

• Please take into account the ambient temperature and the surrounding environment. In addition to ensuring that the room is adequately heated, modify the lighting and music to establish a calming ambiance.

6. **Integrate** Individual Touches:

• Incorporate personalized elements into the massage session. This may encompass the utilization of a specialized massage oil, the inclusion of a preferred fragrance, or the performance of music that carries sentimental significance.

7. Analyze and Test Techniques:

- One may freely explore and determine which massage techniques produce the most favorable results for the partner. This may involve mild stretches, kneading, or even variations of strokes.

8. Requesting Feedback:

- Request feedback throughout the massage session. Verify that your companion is enjoying the experience and is in a comfortable state. This enables real-time adjustments to be implemented.

9. Establish a Relaxing Ambiance:

• Consider the small details that contribute to a tranquil environment. Dim the lighting, fill the space with soothing music, and guarantee that there are no interruptions.

10. A Sensitive Touch:

Have faith in your intuition and observe the body language of your partner. For a pleasant and comfortable experience, adapt your touch in accordance with their reactions.

11. After-Massage Treatment:

• Following the massage, allow your partner some time to unwind. Provide a soothing beverage or a warm towel to augment the post-massage experience.

Conscious communication and attentiveness are fundamental in the process of customizing massages for one another.

Due to the fact that each individual possesses distinct inclinations and sensitivity levels, viewing your partner's cues and feedback with openness will enhance the quality of the experience and make it more enjoyable for all parties.

The Utilization Of Aromatherapy

Aromatherapy can improve the overall experience of a massage by stimulating the sense of smell and encouraging relaxation. The following are some suggestions for incorporating aromatherapy into a massage, particularly with a partner or in a couple setting:

1. Select Aromatherapy-Relaxing Tones:

• Choose essential oils that possess calming properties. Lavender, chamomile, ylang-ylang, and bergamot are typical options. It is said that these fragrances have calming properties.

2. Essential Oil Dilute:

• Prior to topical application, diluted essential oils in a carrier oil are recommended. Coconut oil, jojoba oil, and sweet almond oil are typical carrier oils. This guarantees the safe and effective application of the essential oils onto the skin.

3. Establishing a Relaxing Atmosphere:

• One should employ an essential oil diffuser to impart the desired fragrance into the massage room.

Conversely, a few drops of the essential oil may be applied to a cloth or tissue and positioned throughout the room.

4. Tailor to Specific Individual Preferences:

• Engage in a conversation regarding personal fragrance preferences with your partner. Certain people may have a preference for particular fragrances that they find incredibly calming or pleasurable. Adding a personal touch to the aromatherapy experience through customization.

5. Smell Blending for an Unusual Experience:

• One may engage in the exploration of blending various essential oils in order to generate an unparalleled fragrance. As an illustration, one could blend lavender with a citrus fragrance to create a blend that is both invigorating and soothing.

6. Utilize oil dilution on the skin:

• If your partner has an affinity for direct skin contact, consider dabbing essential oils onto their skin. Concentrate on areas including the neck, wrists, and temples. To prevent skin irritation, use a dilution ratio that is safe to use.

7. Reheat the Oils:

• It is advisable to warm the massage oils prior to their application. This can be accomplished by soaking the oil for several minutes in a bowl of warm water. Warm oils have the ability to heighten one's senses.

8. Employ Aromatherapy Candles to:

• Opt for candles that are infused with essential oils in order to enhance the aesthetic and aromatic qualities of the massage area. Ensure that the candles are positioned securely and away from the massage area.

9. Provision of Aromatherapy Neck Wraps:

• Provide aromatherapy neck wraps or eye pillows with scented herbs or rice. These can be placed over the eyes or around the neck during the massage to enhance relaxation.

10. Discuss Sensitivities:

• Before incorporating aromatherapy, discuss any sensitivities or allergies your partner may have. This ensures that the chosen scents are enjoyable and not irritating.

11. Post-Massage Aromatherapy:

• Extend the aromatherapy experience into the post-massage period. Offer scented towels or a warm aromatherapy bath for continued relaxation.

Remember that individual preferences vary, so it's essential to communicate with your partner about their scent preferences and any potential sensitivities. Aromatherapy can be a delightful addition to a massage, contributing to a multi-sensory and deeply relaxing experience for both individuals involved.

CHAPTER FIVE
Management Of Frequent Obstacles

Although massages can evoke profound relaxation and pleasure, they are not without their share of common obstacles. The following are some suggestions for addressing these challenges:

1. Pain or Discomfort: Resolution: Engage in an open dialogue with the massage therapist regarding your level of discomfort. Should the pressure become unbearable or painful, express your concern without hesitation. The technique of a competent massage therapist will be modified to suit your preferences.

2. Ticklishness: Solution: Inform your massage therapist in advance if you experience ticklishness. One possible adjustment is to employ more forceful pressure or to circumvent excessively delicate regions. Concentrate on deep respiration to assist in reducing ticklish sensations.

3. Adverse Dialogue: Resolution: In the event that one desires a serene and soothing encounter, explicitly inform the massage therapist of this preference prior to the commencement of the session. The majority of clinicians will honor your request for confidentiality.

4. Sensation of Cold or Heat: Resolution: The ideal temperature of the massage chamber may not universally suit all individuals. If you inform the therapist of your level of comfort, they will be able to modify the temperature of the chamber or offer supplementary blankets or fans.

5. Embarrassment or Self-Consciousness: Resolution: A degree of self-consciousness is to be expected, particularly when receiving a massage for the first time. Keep in mind that massage therapists are trained professionals whose primary objective is to ensure a pleasant experience. Inform the therapist in advance of any particular concerns you may have.

6. Difficulty Relaxing: Practice releasing tension while concentrating on your respiration. Please disclose any specific areas in which you are experiencing heightened tension or stress, in order to direct the therapist's attention there.

7. Uncomfortable Positioning: Resolution: Communicate any concerns you may have regarding the bolstering or positioning to the therapist. Adjustments can be made to guarantee your sense of security and relaxation.

8. Post-Massage Soreness: Resolution: Soreness is a frequent occurrence, particularly following a deep tissue massage. Maintain adequate hydration, apply cold or hot compresses when necessary, and inform the therapist if the pressure became unbearable.

9. Residual Oil or Lotion Sensation: Resolution: Consult your therapist if you experience an excessive sensation of oiliness or lotion coverage subsequent to the massage. You may request that they use less oil or furnish you with cloths to remove any surplus.

10. Unanticipated Emotional Release: Resolution: Massage has the potential to elicit emotional reactions on occasion. Accept and communicate your emotions if you find yourself suddenly overcome with emotion. It is an inherent component of the body-mind relationship.

11. Allergic Reactions: Solution: Prefaced notification to the massage therapist of any known allergies or sensitivities to specific oils or lotions is advised.

They may utilize safer alternatives to the products you specify.

Maintaining an open line of communication is crucial in effectively tackling these challenges. Expressing your preferences, concerns, or unexpected reactions to the massage therapist in a vocal manner contributes to the establishment of a positive and comfortable environment that benefits both the client and the therapist.

Suggestions For An Effective Couples Massage

A massage for two people can be an intimate and delightful experience for them to partake in together. The following guidelines will guarantee a successful couple's massage:

1. **Opt for the Appropriate Environment:** Designate a serene and comfortable environment for the massage. This may occur in a retreat, the comfort of one's own residence, or another location renowned for its tranquil ambiance.

2. **Exchange Preferences:** Prior to the massage, negotiate one another's preferences. Discuss specific areas of concentration, the level of duress, and any health concerns or sensitivities that may be present.

3. Establish the Ambiance: Foster a tranquil atmosphere by incorporating subdued lighting, calming music, and potentially fragrant candles or essential oils. The surroundings ought to foster an atmosphere of serenity.

4. Commence the Massage: Commence the massage by performing a mild warm-up. Increase pressure progressively while employing broad strokes to prime the muscles for more intense work.

5. Attempt to Sync Your Movements: If both you and your companion are at ease, attempt to synchronize your movements. This may result in a harmonious experience as the two of you alter positions or move in tandem.

6. Value Boundaries: Demonstrate regard for one another's personal space and limits. Throughout the massage, verify that your companion is at ease with the pressure and techniques being applied.

7. Technique Experimentation: Do not hesitate to engage in the exploration of various massage techniques. Explore the combination of kneading, mild stretches, and strokes to determine which one feels most comfortable for you both.

8. Employ Premium Massage Products: Select massage oils or moisturizers of superior quality. If both of you appreciate fragrant products, consider using them for aromatherapy; however, be mindful of any sensitivities or allergies.

9. Temperature Observance: Maintain a comfortable temperature in the chamber. Provide additional comforters or towels in order to accommodate individual preferences.

10. It is advisable to maintain an open line of communication throughout the massage. Inform your partner if something causes them discomfort or thrills them unusually. It enriches the experience that is shared.

11. Rotate companions: When receiving and providing massages, alternate companions so that each individual can experience the benefits to the fullest. Because it is a collaborative endeavor, both participants should experience a sense of concern.

12. Post-Massage Relaxation: Allow time for relaxation following the massage. Offer your companion a resting area that is conducive to comfort, as well as water or a calming beverage to ensure proper hydration.

13. Exchange Feedback: Following the massage, exchange your views and feedback with one another. Discuss what went well and whether any modifications are necessary for future endeavors.

14. Post-massage Proposal: Arrange a leisurely activity or a period of companionship following the massage.

Prolonged periods of relaxation, such as sharing an intimate dinner, bathing, or embracing, have the potential to elevate the overall experience.

It is imperative to bear in mind that effective couples massage relies on communication, mutual respect, and the establishment of a positive and tranquil environment.

Adapt the experience to the preferences of both companions, and savor the moments of connection and relaxation that are shared.

CHAPTER SIX
Expert Assistance And Continuing Education

Seeking professional assistance and pursuing continuing education are critical components for massage therapists to uphold a prosperous and gratifying profession. The following are methods by which massage therapists can obtain expert assistance and engage in ongoing educational endeavors:

• **Mentorship and Supervision:** Participate in mentorship and supervision programs led by seasoned massage therapists or healthcare experts. This facilitates the provision of guidance, feedback, and knowledge exchange.

• Belonging to professional massage therapy associations and organizations is recommended. Resources, networking opportunities, and access to conferences and seminars are frequently provided by these organizations.

• **Participation in Workshops and Seminars:** Regularly attend conferences, seminars, and workshops to remain informed about the most recent industry trends, research, and techniques. These events afford invaluable opportunities to gain knowledge from subject matter authorities.

• **Certifications and Specializations:** Advanced certifications and specializations in particular massage modalities or techniques should be pursued. By doing so, one not only improves their skill set but also showcases a dedication to ongoing professional growth.

•   **Peer Collaboration:** Share knowledge and experiences through collaboration with peers and colleagues. Peer learning has the potential to yield significant insights and pragmatic advice.

• **Clinical Conferences:** Participate in clinical conferences that pertain to the fields of healthcare, wellness, and massage therapy. These conferences frequently attract eminent lecturers and practical sessions that aim to enhance the knowledge of practitioners on a wide range of subjects.

- **Literature and Journals:** By reading books, research articles, and journals that pertain to the disciplines of allied health and massage therapy. Maintaining awareness of industry literature and current research is an asset to the implementation of evidence-based practice.

- **Advanced Training Institutes:** Investigate training centers and institutes that are specifically dedicated to advanced massage therapy techniques. These institutions frequently provide all-encompassing programs designed to enhance one's skill set.

- **Personal Professional Development Plans:** Construct an individual professional development plan that delineates precise objectives pertaining to the acquisition of knowledge, certifications, and skill improvement. Review and revise this plan frequently in order to monitor progress.

- **Participation in Therapist Support Groups or Forums:** For individuals seeking guidance, establish connections with fellow professionals, and exchange personal experiences, consider joining therapist support groups or forums. Local or online organizations can offer encouragement and a sense of community.

- **Engagement in Consultation with Healthcare Professionals:** Foster interprofessional learning by collaborating with healthcare professionals, including physical therapists and chiropractors. By doing so, the therapist's comprehension of complementary healthcare practices may be expanded.

- **Integral Competencies:** For a comprehensive repertoire that surpasses mere proficiency in massage techniques, enroll in academic programs that cover business management, ethics, and effective communication.

- Prioritize self-care practices in order to preserve one's physical and mental health. This could encompass engaging in routine physical activity, practicing mindfulness, and participating in pursuits that promote a harmonious equilibrium between work and personal life.

Continuing education is essential not only for skill maintenance and improvement, but also for keeping abreast of industry developments and best practices. It exhibits a dedication to maintaining a professional demeanor and prioritizing the welfare of clients. Moreover, in order to sustain a prosperous and viable profession in massage therapy, it is critical to seek professional assistance when necessary, including for career guidance or mental health support.

Summary

Massage therapy is a multifaceted and gratifying discipline that incorporates an extensive array of methods with the objective of fostering both physical and mental health.

Enhanced overall benefits can be obtained from both massage therapists and individuals desiring massages through knowledge of the various modalities, the significance of effective communication, and the ability to personalize experiences.

Ongoing professional development, seeking mentorship, and remaining informed about industry trends are all factors that contribute to the achievement of success and satisfaction in the field of massage therapy.

By maintaining up-to-date knowledge on emerging research and methodologies and integrating sophisticated techniques, therapists can guarantee the delivery of exceptional care to their clients.

Promoting mindfulness during the massage session, fostering effective communication with the therapist, and establishing a comfortable environment are all factors that can contribute to a more pleasurable and therapeutic experience for the recipient.

The key to creating a memorable experience, whether for two people or one, is to customize the massage to the individual's preferences and requirements.

It is important to bear in mind that massage therapy encompasses more than mere muscle manipulation; rather, it employs a holistic approach that takes into account the interplay between the mind and body. In addition to promoting relaxation and reducing tension, massage can also be utilized to treat specific musculoskeletal conditions.

In the ongoing development of massage therapy, the active

participation of both practitioners and clients is crucial in influencing and deriving advantages from this time-honored and therapeutic modality. The objective of both providing and receiving massages is to enhance the quality of life and promote overall well-being.

THE END

www.ingramcontent.com/pod-product-compliance
Lightning Source LLC
Chambersburg PA
CBHW071601270726
48661CB00017B/339